20 Questions and Answers About Shift Work Disorder

Sudhansu Chokroverty, MD, FRCP, FACP

Professor and Co-Chair of Neurology
Program Director of Clinical Neurophysiology & Sleep Medicine
New Jersey Neuroscience Institute at JFK Medical Center
Seton Hall University
Edison, NJ

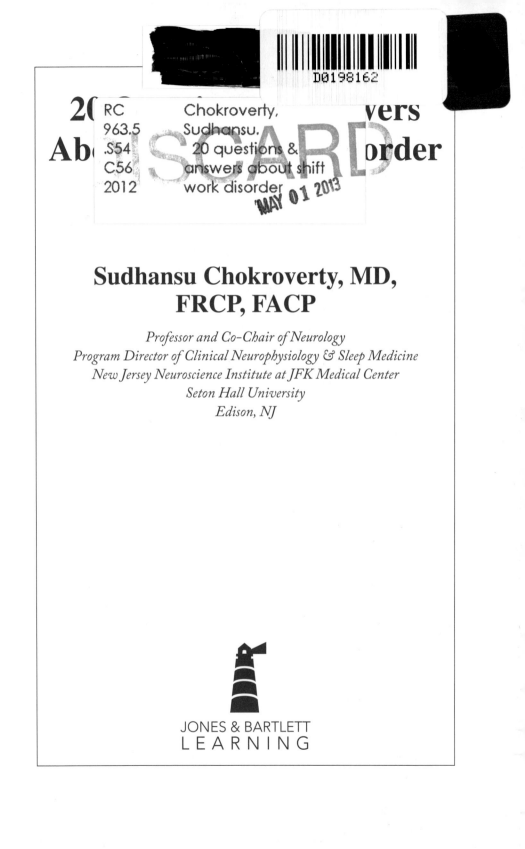

JONES & BARTLETT
LEARNING

World Headquarters

Jones & Bartlett Learning
40 Tall Pine Drive
Sudbury, MA 01776
978-443-5000
info@jblearning.com
www.jblearning.com

Jones & Bartlett Learning
Canada
6339 Ormindale Way
Mississauga, Ontario L5V 1J2
Canada

Jones & Bartlett Learning
International
Barb House, Barb Mews
London W6 7PA
United Kingdom

Jones & Bartlett Learning books and products are available through most bookstores and online booksellers. To contact Jones & Bartlett Learning directly, call 800-832-0034, fax 978-443-8000, or visit our website, www.jblearning.com.

Substantial discounts on bulk quantities of Jones & Bartlett Learning publications are available to corporations, professional associations, and other qualified organizations. For details and specific discount information, contact the special sales department at Jones & Bartlett Learning via the above contact information or send an email to specialsales@jblearning.com.

The authors, editor, and publisher have made every effort to provide accurate information. However, they are not responsible for errors, omissions, or for any outcomes related to the use of the contents of this book and take no responsibility for the use of the products and procedures described. Treatments and side effects described in this book may not be applicable to all people; likewise, some people may require a dose or experience a side effect that is not described herein. Drugs and medical devices are discussed that may have limited availability controlled by the Food and Drug Administration (FDA) for use only in a research study or clinical trial. Research, clinical practice, and government regulations often change the accepted standard in this field. When consideration is being given to use of any drug in the clinical setting, the healthcare provider or reader is responsible for determining FDA status of the drug, reading the package insert, and reviewing prescribing information for the most up-to-date recommendations on dose, precautions, and contraindications, and determining the appropriate usage for the product. This is especially important in the case of drugs that are new or seldom used.

Production Credits
Executive Publisher: Christopher Davis
Managing Editor, Special Projects:
  Kathy Richardson
Associate Production Editor: Leah Corrigan
Associate Marketing Manager: Katie Hennessey
Manufacturing and Inventory Control
  Supervisor: Amy Bacus

Composition: Lynn L'Heureux
Cover Design: Kristin Parker
Cover Images: (from left) © Showface/
  Dreamstime.com, © Martindata/
  Dreamstime.com, © Rmarmion/Dreamstime.
  com, © Crystal Craig/Dreamstime.com
Printing and Binding: Malloy, Inc.
Cover Printing: Malloy, Inc.

ISBN-978-1-4496-2100-1

6048

Printed in the United States of America
14 13 12 11 10   10 9 8 7 6 5 4 3 2 1

CONTENTS

Part 2: Shift Work Disorder   *19*

Shift work (SW) has created a modern paradox. On one hand it has increased profit and productivity of the society; on the other hand SW has generated its own adverse effects by challenging our internal body clock located deep in the brain to rapidly adjust to Earth's geophysical environment thereby creating a mismatch between internal and external time keepers. This results in serious adverse consequences in the form of excessive sleepiness under inappropriate circumstances and in inappropriate places or insomnia in some susceptible individuals. The end result is shift work disorder (SWD), which may cause short-term and long-term undesirable consequences. We must deal with this either by adjusting the shifts or by other non-pharmacological and pharmacological means. In a question and answer format in this booklet I tried to summarize briefly the concepts of SW, SWD, their consequences, diagnosis, and treatment to heighten public awareness about shift work, a necessary inconvenience of modern industrialized society.

ACKNOWLEDGMENTS

First I must express my appreciation to my wife, Manisha Chokroverty, MD, for her unfailing encouragement, support, and patience during the preparation of this book during our mini vacation.

I wish to thank Betty Coram for typing the entire booklet, Annabella Drennan for corrections of the proofs, and Jenny Rodriguez for some help with typing. Special thanks are due to Christopher Davis, Executive Publisher, Medicine, Kathy Richardson, and Leah Corrigan at Jones & Bartlett Learning for their professionalism and dedication. Finally, I must thank Bindi and Staci for allowing us to include their version as patients.

PART ONE

Shift Work

Q1. What is shift work and what are different types of shifts?

Thomas Edison's invention of the light bulb in 1879 created a change in society that impacts us to this day. Historically, the usual sleeping hours for mankind were a few hours after sunset and before sunrise. During prehistoric civilization there were two periods of sleep: the first sleep of about four hours with a middle-of-the-night break for chores, intimacy and other activities; the second sleep for about another four hours. After the invention of the light bulb people were able to work at night, laying the groundwork for our current society of a 24/7 world with increased productivity and changing lifestyles. This shift of work schedule from traditional daytime (9 to 5) to untraditional night time or rotating between night and day is known as **shift work** (i.e., shifting the work schedule outside traditional working hours). It is estimated that shift work is performed by about 20% (over 15,000,000) of working people in the USA and Western Europe. Unfortunately, this shift in work schedule disrupts the normal human sleep-wake pattern and the body's **circadian rhythm**, sometimes causing undesirable consequences.

Shift work

Untraditional night or rotating between night and day work schedule.

Circadian rhythm

Internal body clock representing a 24-hour cycle.

The number of shift workers in both industrialized and developing nations is rising by perhaps about 3% to 4% each year due to companies' efforts to increase profit and productivity in manufacturing industries. Shift work has long been traditional in law enforcement and the armed forces. In addition, service industries like restaurants and convenience stores tend to remain open much longer than normal business hours. Workers in fields related to public safety, transportation, and health care, (e.g., police, fire fighters, air traffic controllers, security, emergency medical transportation, hospitals [interns and residents, nurses and other workers]), and those working at energy power plants or the maritime industry (e.g., fishing vessels) all regularly participate in shift work as part of normal business operations. The national weather service and private weather forecasting companies utilize shift work to constantly monitor the weather. In addition, "call centers" overseas and much of the Internet service industry depend heavily on shift work. Other occupations requiring shift work include entertainment and hospitality (performers, radio DJs, bartenders, and doormen). While these industries all benefit from the flexibility of shift workers, the change in schedule can have undesirable short- and long-term consequences for some workers.

There are different types of nontraditional work shifts: grave-yard or night shift (10 pm to 6 am); early morning shift (6 am to 2 pm); and late afternoon to early evening shift (2 pm to 10 pm). Shifts can be permanent, fixed, or rotating. Shifts can rotate forward (clockwise) (e.g., from morning to evening to night time) or backward (e.g., night to afternoon to early morning shift). Rotating shifts cause more sleep dif-ficulties than permanent shifts and counterclockwise rotation negatively affects sleep-wake activities more than clockwise rotation. In addition to direction of rotation, the speed of rotation can be slow or rapid and the length of the shift may also vary; all of these factors (see Question 4) can affect your sleep-wake schedule and impact your feelings of fatigue and wakefulness. An example of a rapidly rotating shift is to work 2–3 days in a row on a particular shift, followed by 2–3 days of work on a different shift. An example of a slowly rotating shift is working 5–7 days in a row on a particular shift and then rotating 2 days off before another shift. Rapidly rotating shifts result in fewer sleep hours than slowly rotating shifts. The two most common shift lengths are 8 hours and 12 hours; the lat-ter is common among workers on oil rigs and at healthcare facilities and nuclear power plants. Fatigue and wakefulness are significant concerns during 12-hour shifts.

Shifts can rotate forward (clockwise) (e.g., from morning to evening to night time) or backward (e.g., night to afternoon to early morning shift).

Q2. How does shift work affect the sleep–wake cycle and other body rhythms?

Every living cell has a rhythm. For example, our sleep-wake habit follows a circadian (from the Latin *circa*, meaning "about" and *dian*, meaning "day") rhythm. Shift work disrupts our circadian rhythm, which is controlled by an internal clock located in a part of the brain called the hypothalamus. This special center regulates appetite, hormone secretion, water intake, temperature, and sleep-wake cycles. The human internal clock is thought to reside within a cluster of nerve cells that receive signals from the retina (the layer of nerve cells in the back of the eye responsible for transmitting visual images). This internal clock is connected to multiple parts of the body—not only the retina for receiving light from the outside world, but also other parts of the nervous system, which allows it to control several functions. Environmental (outside) light helps us to complete our circadian timing system (circadian rhythm) to a 24-hour day.

Our sleep-wake habits are controlled not only by external light and darkness (as determined by sunrise and sunset), but also by our internal body clock.

Our sleep-wake habits are controlled not only by external light and darkness (as determined by sunrise and sunset), but also by our internal body clock. This was proven more than two and a half centuries ago by a French astronomer named de Mairan. He noticed that the leaves of a certain plant (heliotrope) would open at sunrise and close at sunset, even when the plant was kept inside, away from sunlight. This observation led de Mairan to conclude that an internal clock in the plant must control the opening and closing of the leaves. Only in 1972 did scientists discover the existence of a similar internal clock in rats. Shortly thereafter, researchers confirmed that such a clock operates in humans as well.

Experiments have been conducted to isolate humans from all external sources of time cues (for example, by having subjects live in bunkers, caves, or a special laboratory environment). In these investigations, the individuals had no idea about sunrise, sunset, light, darkness, time of day, or time for meals. They did not have a clock, telephone, or television. They were allowed to sleep, wake up, and eat whenever they wanted. Under these circumstances (called "free running rhythm", because the body's internal clock is not synchronized with the environmental time), the length of the human day appears to be a little longer than 24 hours (close to 24.2 hours).

When our internal clock is in conflict with "outside" time as shown on a wristwatch or clock, all rhythms (sleep-wake, temperature, and hormone secretion) become desynchronized, thus disrupting our normal circadian rhythm. Such disruption is very common in shift workers, particularly night shift workers. In such a case, the internal body clock does not match the external clock, which gives time according to sunrise and sunset. Our brains make note of external cues that tell us to be awake (sunlight, time on a clock, other people up and about), but for shift workers this is often the very time of day they need to sleep. This disruption of the circadian rhythm can cause serious sleep disturbances and undesirable consequences (see Question 5).

As stated in Question 1, shift work means working outside the traditional hours. As a result, we force ourselves to stay awake when our body clock tells us to go to sleep. For example, a night shift worker is supposed to stay awake at night when he is used to sleeping. In contrast, our circadian rhythm puts pressure on us to remain wakeful in the morning and early afternoon, but night shift workers must sleep during those hours. The schedule is also disrupted in workers during other types of shifts. This is how shift work affects sleep-wake and other body rhythms, causing a number of short- and long-term consequences (see Question 5). This mismatch between our internal clock controlling sleep-wake and other rhythms and the external clock (environment) creates some serious confusion in our natural body rhythms, requiring shift workers to adapt their bodies to a new schedule. People have differing amounts of success in adapting to a schedule change, based on a number of factors (see Question 4).

Our sleep-wake schedule is driven by two opposing forces: our circadian rhythm controlled by an internal master clock (see above), which affects the timing of sleep and a **homeostatic sleep drive** that controls sleep intensity and is determined by how long we have been awake. These two processes work in harmony to determine our sleep-wake schedule. At night, close to our individual bedtime, homeostatic pressure increases and

Homeostatic sleep drive

The desire to sleep that gradually increases with prolonged wakefulness.

5

circadian force fades, resulting in peaceful sleep. There are two periods in a 24 hour cycle when we have the strongest desire to sleep: mid-afternoon between 3 and 5 pm and again in the early morning hours between 3 and 5 am, when our body temperature is at its lowest point. The two most significant problems with shift work are excessive sleepiness during work at night and the inability to have good quality restorative sleep during non-working hours. Most of the other consequences result from these two major symptoms. Approximately 70% of shift workers occasionally complain of these two symptoms, but when these become excessive and intense, interfering with function, shift work disorder occurs (see Question 13).

Q3. Why does shift work cause adverse effects on health?

Shift work causes a circadian mismatch of a person's normal sleep-wake schedule, which can sometimes result in excessive sleepiness during undesirable times (e.g., at work) or not enough restorative sleep during non-working hours to function effectively. Some experts believe that those workers on permanent night shift sleep 1 to 4 hours less and those on rotation shifts sleep 2 to 2 1/2 hours less than day workers. Night shift workers average about 6 hours of sleep and those on rotating shifts sleep about 5 1/2 hours. This amount of sleep is less than what regular daytime workers normally achieve. There are several reasons for this reduced amount of sleep. For one thing, shift workers must attempt to sleep at a time when their circadian or wakefulness drive is exerting pressure to remain awake (e.g., morning or early afternoon for night shift workers). In addition, the desire to spend some quality time with family or take care of other household or social obligations, and a home environment not conducive to sleep (e.g., noise, light, telephone rings, other people working in the kitchen or next door, etc.) are obstacles to adequate sleep. Chronic sleep deficit (not achieving enough sleep each night)—for shift workers or due to any other reason—has been shown in various studies to cause many adverse long-term symptoms. These include higher rates of illness (and even death) as well as increased rates of high blood pressure, coronary arterial disease, diabetes mellitus, and obesity (see Question 5).

The other major effect is excessive sleepiness and fatigue at work due to a combination of an inadequate amount of sleep during the daytime (night shift workers' usual sleep period) and increasing sleep pressure accumulating during the nighttime. This excessive sleepiness at work combined with unrefreshing sleep during off hours make these workers vulnerable to accidents at work and while commuting home in the morning, creating major public and personal safety issues (see Question 5). On days off, shift workers often try to change back to their normal sleep-wake schedule, which further worsens their sleep quality. Finally, all the physiological rhythms of the body are altered by not getting enough sleep—those affecting almost every system, including the endocrine system, which is responsible for the secretion of various hormones and chemicals. The endocrine system helps regulate your mood, tissue function, and your metabolism. Therefore, decreased quality and quantity of sleep coupled with altered physiological rhythms may cause a variety of long-term medical consequences and safety-related issues (see Question 5).

Q4. What factors influence the effect of shift work on sleep and wakefulness?

The effect that shift work can have on sleep and wakefulness is determined by several factors. Sleep problems in shift workers are mainly due to disruption of the normal sleep-wake rhythm. The two most important problems are excessive sleepiness during work at night (for night shift workers) and an inability to maintain good quality restorative sleep during non-working hours in the daytime. Most of the other consequences (see Question 5) result from these two major symptoms. While most shift workers complain of these two symptoms at one time or another, it is when these symptoms become excessive

The two most important problems are excessive sleepiness during work at night (for night shift workers) and an inability to maintain good quality restorative sleep during non-working hours in the daytime.

and occur too frequently that workers are thought to be suffering from shift work disorder.

Table 1 provides a list of factors that can play a significant role in determining whether a shift work schedule will have a strong impact on someone's sleep and wakefulness cycles.

Table 1. Factors Influencing Effects of Shift Work on Sleep and Wakefulness

- Types of shifts (e.g., permanent, rotating)
- Duration of shift
- Speed of rotation (slow or fast)
- Direction of rotation (clockwise or counterclockwise)
- Psychological stress
- Social and family disruption
- Coping mechanisms
- Fatigue
- Unknown biological mechanism
- Exposure to light (natural or artificial)
- Existing health problems
- Age (over 50 is more adversely affected than younger people)
- Gender (female shift workers have more difficulty coping with the stress of shift work than men)

There are different types of shifts and rotations (see Question 1), all of which may have negative effects on sleep and wakefulness. Some research studies have found that rotating shifts (e.g., day to evening to night shifts) result in equal amounts of sleep duration (how long you sleep) for those working on permanent night shifts, but most studies found that total sleep in night shift workers (about six hours) is less than that in evening and slowly rotating shift workers. Those workers on a rotating shift schedule get less sleep after a night shift compared with permanent night shift workers because of the ability to adjust to working at night. Rapidly rotating shifts (e.g., 2 to 3 days in a row in one shift followed by 2–3 days off or working on a different type of shift) result in less sleep than slowly rotating shifts (e.g., 5–7 days in a row followed by 2–3 days off using at least 2 weeks per shift schedule). Clockwise (forward) rotation is similar to something called "phase delay" or what happens when you travel westward (the days are longer). Counterclockwise (backward) rotation, on the other hand, is similar to phase advance or traveling eastward (the days are shorter). Your body clock (circadian clock) adjusts better to clockwise rotation because it is naturally easier to delay sleep to a later hour and so this has a less severe effect on sleep. In addition, findings from several studies show that shifts that last 10–12 hours compared with 8-hour shifts cause more sleepiness and a greater risk of accidents.

Fatigue and wakefulness are of particular concern during 12-hour shifts. It is important to differentiate fatigue from sleepiness. Fatigue is physical or mental exhaustion or tiredness that can be triggered by factors such as stress, medication, overwork, or mental and physical illness or disease. Sleepiness is the body's tendency to fall asleep. One way of differentiating between the two is that if you had the opportunity to fall asleep in a comfortable, sleep-conducive environment, you would readily fall asleep if you were suffering from sleepiness, but not if you were suffering just from fatigue. Another difference is that physical and mental fatigue may be reduced by resting or relaxing, but this will just make sleepiness worse. Furthermore, people show tell-tale signs of sleepiness such as a feeling of heaviness and drooping of the eyelids, nodding of the head, and reduced blinking, but do not display any clear signs of fatigue. Other factors that affect the influence of shift work schedules are age and sex. Adaptation to shift work is more difficult for older workers (around 50 years or older) than for younger workers. Typically, women doing shift work get less sleep than men because of their increased family and social obligations.

Fatigue is physical or mental exhaustion or tiredness that can be triggered by factors such as stress, medication, overwork, or mental and physical illness or disease.

Q5. What are the short-term and long-term consequences of shift work?

Short-term consequences of shift work result from shift workers' sleep disturbance as well as the psychological stress of shift work (see **Table 2**). These consequences are more intense in those suffering from shift work disorder (see Question 13). Many studies have shown a negative effect on performance and safety related to sleepiness and sleep disturbance in shift workers and individuals with shift work disorder. Research studies have clearly shown an increased number of occurrences of accidents at work and during the commute home from work, specifically for night shift workers, as well as when they are driving on other occasions. Impaired productivity and performance with increasing work-related errors, absenteeism, and sick leave are some of the short-term consequences seen in some shift workers and those suffering from shift work disorder. The other short-term consequences include disrupted social and family life, not enough time with spouse and children (which can cause severe psychological stress), and social isolation, all of which may contribute to an increased possibility of developing depression (see Question 12), alcohol abuse, or nicotine addiction (smoking) in some shift work disorder patients.

Many people, after months or years of shift work, will develop shift work disorder and other serious long-term negative consequences (see Table 2). Some of the illnesses listed in Table 2 are associated directly with shift work, whereas others are associated with symptoms of insomnia and excessive sleepiness related to shift work disorder. These consequences are greatest among patients with shift work disorder and not all shift workers will experience these. So far, studies have given conflicting results regarding why and how often these consequences occur, so a definite conclusion regarding the connection between shift work and these consequences cannot be made just yet. We do know that after many years of shift work, some individuals, even after leaving the job,

Impaired productivity and performance with increasing work-related errors, absenteeism, and sick leave are some of the short-term consequences seen in some shift workers and those suffering from shift work disorder.

will be left with **chronic sleep disturbance** (inability to get enough good quality sleep resulting in daytime sleepiness). The likelihood that this will occur may depend on individual personality, coping mechanism, persistent depression, family problems, possible divorce, and other individual factors.

Chronic sleep disturbance

The inability to obtain sufficient amount of good quality sleep resulting in daytime sleepiness.

Table 2. Potential Short-Term and Long-Term Consequences of Shift Work

Potential short-term consequences

- Sleep disturbance (excessive sleepiness at work or an inability to obtain good quality sleep during sleep period)
- Impaired performance and productivity at work
- Absenteeism and sick leave
- Sleepiness-related accidents at work and while commuting home from work and on other occasions
- Disruption in social and family life

Potential long-term consequences

- Chronic sleep disturbance
- Gastrointestinal problems including peptic ulcers
- Cardiovascular disorders
- Increased occurrence of type II diabetes mellitus
- Increased body mass index (obesity)
- Metabolic problems (e.g., high blood cholesterol and triglyceride levels)
- High blood pressure
- Increased prevalence of certain cancers
- Depression
- Impaired quality of life
- Undesirable pregnancy outcomes (this remains unproven)
- Increased morbidity and mortality

Shift Work

11

20 QUESTIONS & ANSWERS ABOUT SHIFT WORK DISORDER

Gastrointestinal symptoms (see Question 8) and ulcers are more frequent in shift workers who experience insomnia or excessive sleepiness and these symptoms may also be related to shift work itself. The risk of heart disease is most probably related to the shift work rather than to symptoms of insomnia or excessive sleepiness. The increased risk of cardiovascular disease, however, could be related to chronic loss of sleep hours (sleep deficit) rather than a shift in circadian cycle.

Several studies have indicated that over time, the effect of a shift worker's body metabolism becoming out of sync can result in an increased risk of diabetes, obesity and its associated consequences (e.g., heart disease, high blood pressure, coronary arterial disease, sleep apnea), and elevated blood cholesterol and triglyceride levels. Some studies indicate that after many years of shift work there may be an increased risk for certain cancers (e.g., breast and endometrial cancers in women, non-Hodgkin lymphoma, and prostate cancer in men [see Question 9]). Long-term psychological stress related to shift work, coupled with chronic sleep deprivation, impaired quality of sleep and in certain cases, disruption of family and social life and divorce, resulted in depression in some shift workers. There is some weak evidence that shift work in women may lead to undesirable pregnancy outcomes (such as increased miscarriage rates, premature deliveries, reduced birth weight of babies). Some studies have linked night shift work in nurses with other negative women's health issues such as irregular menstruation and reduced ability to get pregnant. Several studies have shown an increased mortality rate in shift workers but the cause is uncertain and may be related to long-term sleep deprivation, increased use of alcohol and hypnotic medications, and smoking.

Long-term psychological stress related to shift work, coupled with chronic sleep deprivation, impaired quality of sleep and in certain cases, disruption of family and social life and divorce, resulted in depression in some shift workers.

Q6. What is the "social cost" of shift work?

There are numerous public safety and "social cost" issues related to shift work and these affect family, friends, the community, and the worker's own sense of well-being. There are both literal and figurative costs related to shift work. For example, fatigue at work may lead to decreased attention to detail, possibly resulting in occupational accidents. These accidents can be minor or significant, such as a near melt-down at a nuclear power plant, a chemical explosion, train derailment, shuttle disaster, or an oil spill. Other safety issues include auto accidents while commuting or even on days off. These events cost society billions of dollars and thousands of lives. The rare, the dramatic, and the frequent small events all result from poor performance on the part of the shift worker due to fatigue, poor concentration, and tiredness. These symptoms are exacerbated by multiple factors, including sleep disturbance, social and family disruption, and psychological stress.

Q7. My friend told me that shift work may exacerbate or cause heart disease and high blood pressure. Is my friend correct?

Your friend may very well be correct. However, study results have been somewhat mixed and controversial. Research has yet to determine whether the increased rate of heart disease and high blood pressure is directly related to shift work, is a result of chronic sleep deprivation, or if there are other unknown and related factors. Further research is therefore needed. There is certainly a slight indication that shift workers experience higher rates of heart disease and high blood pressure, but evidence as to the exact cause is not yet conclusive.

Researchers assume that the connection between heart disease and shift work is based on a combination of behavioral, psychosocial, and physiological factors. Behavioral factors include work-related stress and balancing of family life and work. Psychosocial factors consist of sleep disturbance, increased smoking and alcohol consumption, weight gain, inadequate nutrition, and physical inactivity. Physiological factors include

Shift Work

activation of the autonomic nervous system (the part of the nervous system that controls blood circulation and breathing) causing increased heart rate, high blood pressure, and irregular hormone secretion; thickening of the blood vessels; and metabolic changes in the body (for example weight gain and high cholesterol) to diabetes. For now, research studies have given conflicting results, but the connection continues to be studied.

Q8. One of my relatives has been working on the night shift for five years. He recently consulted a physician for peptic ulcer and other gastrointestinal symptoms. Could this be related to shift work?

It is difficult to determine if your relative's symptoms are directly related to his work schedule. However, it has long been recognized that shift workers are at increased risk for gastrointestinal symptoms and peptic ulcer disease. As stated in Question 5, this association could be due to both sleep disturbance and shift work itself. It has been suggested that shift workers are at increased risk for gastroduodenal ulcers (lesions or sores in the lining of the stomach or small intestine) due to increased release of certain hormones in the stomach (gastrin and pepsinogen). It is possible that the increased release of these hormones is due to the sleep disturbance that shift workers experience. Several other factors, such as smoking, age, alteration of normal eating habits (especially on the night shift), and socioeconomic status must be taken into consideration in future studies before a firm conclusion can be made about the connection between shift work and gastrointestinal disease.

Q9. My friend has been working on nights or rotating shifts in a chemical plant. She read on the Internet that she may be in danger of developing cancer. Is my friend correct?

There are many studies linking long-term shift work with increased rates of certain types of cancers, although the evidence is not convincing yet. In 2007, the World Health Organization (WHO) announced that overnight shift work that "involves circadian disruption" would be classified as a "probable" cause of cancer. Increased risk of developing breast and endometrial (the lining of the uterus) cancers in women, prostate cancer in men, colorectal cancer, and non-Hodgkin's lymphoma have been noted based on several studies. In some studies the conclusions and findings are simply based on looking at annual health check-up files for certain types of shift workers and considering the numbers of years they have spent doing shift work. Other studies used simple questionnaires and did not consider types and duration of shifts. Furthermore, a few studies generated negative findings (that is, there was no association between cancer and shift work). Despite various weaknesses in the designs of some studies, as well as those producing negative results, the general tentative conclusion is that there is probable cause for concern regarding an association between long-term (20 years or more) shift work and cancer, but further research is needed to be certain. The explanations for how and why cancer and shift work are linked are complicated and involve many factors. One possible suggestion for female shift workers developing breast cancer is that their increased exposure to artificial (indoor) lighting at night causes their bodies to cut back on producing melatonin (a hormone). Without enough melatonin, there women's levels of estrogen go up, which in turn might cause an increase in circulating estrogen—a hormone that has been linked to breast cancer.

Q10. I am a sleep technologist who has been working on the night shift three nights per week for the past three years. At the beginning, I had mild sleepiness on the job but I managed to overcome it by following good sleep hygiene measures. Lately I have been experiencing uncontrollable sleepiness on the job. My husband also told me that my snoring has become louder than before. What has been happening to me?

Before your healthcare provider can accurately answer this question and suggest recommendations, s/he needs to know the answers to several questions. Did you change your shift from fixed to rotating? Did you change shift duration? Did you change your place of work, requiring a longer commuting distance? Do you have any recent health issues, for example, a medical or neurological disorder or a psychiatric problem causing depression? Did you gain weight recently? Is your snoring loud and frequent enough to disturb your husband's sleep? Has your husband noticed that you stop breathing from time to time during your sleep? If you suffer from a new medical, neurological, or psychiatric (such as anxiety or depression) disorder, these may impact your sleep, causing you to have excessive sleepiness. From the description, it appears that you may be developing sleep apnea, especially if you have been snoring loudly almost daily and if you have gained weight. Sleep apnea is common and often under-diagnosed or undiagnosed. Common symptoms of sleep apnea include disturbed sleep and snoring, temporary stopping of breathing during sleep, and excessive daytime sleepiness. It is more common in middle-aged or elderly men but becomes increasingly prevalent in women during their postmenopausal years. Contact your healthcare provider, who will most likely refer you to a sleep specialist to confirm the diagnosis after adequate history and physical examination, along with laboratory tests

Sleep apnea is common and often under-diagnosed or undiagnosed.

of overnight sleep recording (see Question 17). It is important to confirm a diagnosis of sleep apnea, as there is effective treatment to prevent short-term and long-term consequences (such as heart failure, high blood pressure, stroke, memory impairment, diabetes mellitus).

Q11. I am a 32-year-old nurse suffering from narcolepsy which is currently well controlled on medication. About 6 months ago, I began to work night shifts at the hospital. Since then, my narcoleptic symptoms have gone out of control. Could it be due to shift work?

The worsening of your narcoleptic symptoms shortly after starting shift work is most probably related to your new schedule. A prominent symptom of **narcolepsy** is uncontrollable or excessive sleepiness that occurs in inappropriate places and under inappropriate circumstances. These excessive symptoms are generally well controlled after taking wake-promoting or stimulant medication. By changing your work to non-traditional hours you are now disrupting your sleep-wake schedule, which adds to the burden of sleepiness caused by narcolepsy and worsens your symptoms. There may be additional reasons (see Question 10) for this increase in symptoms. Therefore, you should consult your healthcare provider for a correct diagnosis and further recommendations for treatment.

Staci writes:

*I am a registered nurse and have been working on permanent night shifts (7 pm to 7 am) three nights a week for the past eight years. I have experienced excessive daytime sleepiness since childhood and in 2008 underwent a surgical procedure to resect a pituitary tumor (prolactinoma). Based on my symptoms and findings from PSG and MSLT tests (see Question 17) performed in December 2008, I was diagnosed with narcolepsy. Except for excessive sleepiness and occasional **sleep paralysis**, I did not have other symptoms of narcolepsy, such as **cataplexy** or vivid frightening dreams. Working 12*

Narcolepsy

Chronic neurological sleep disorder characterized by overwhelming daytime drowsiness and sudden attacks of sleep.

Sleep paralysis

The inability to voluntarily move when falling asleep or waking up.

Cataplexy

A sudden loss of muscle tone and strength without loss of consciousness.

hours overnight for the past eight years has had a profound impact on my sleep cycle. The commute home can be quite long due to traffic and feels even longer when compounded by my body's desire to sleep right then and there. Even when I am extremely tired from being up overnight, I can sometimes only achieve 2–4 hours of continuous sleep at most. Some days I cannot sleep at all and remain awake until it is time to get ready for work again. On my nights off, I wake up 2–3 hours after going to sleep. Some nights I can go back to sleep, but on others I stay awake until the early morning. Even though night shift work has such negative effects on my sleeping time, there are no plans for me to change to a day shift worker. In the past I had some success with taking wake-promoting medication for excessive sleepiness with some benefit, but sleep medications for insomnia were not much help.

Q12. I am a 50-year-old woman who has worked on permanent night shifts at the hospital for the past three years. I have recently started experiencing mood swings. Am I developing shift work related depression?

This is an important question and should be settled after consultation with your healthcare provider. As stated (see Questions 5 and 13), chronic sleep deprivation due to insomnia caused by shift work may lead to later depression. Studies have conclusively shown that there is a two-way relationship between insomnia and depression. That is, patients who suffer from chronic insomnia are prone to develop mood swings (depression) at a later date and depression itself is a risk factor for insomnia. Stated simply, depression can cause insomnia and insomnia can lead to depression. Shift work itself imposes considerable psychiatric stress (see Questions 3 and 5) for a variety of reasons, such as sleep disturbance, disruption of family and social life, insufficient quality time spent with children and spouse, job stress, and other factors.

PART TWO

Shift Work Disorder

Q13. What is shift work disorder?

Some shift workers cannot successfully adapt to the disruption of their sleep-wake cycle, due to some unknown individual factor, and they develop symptoms of shift work disorder. It should be noted that the vast majority of shift workers can never completely adapt to permanent night or rotating shifts but somehow manage to cope with the changing schedule. In those individuals who are prone to develop symptoms of shift work disorder, the coping mechanisms break down. The two most important complaints in shift work disorder are excessive sleepiness in working hours and an inability to fall asleep or initiate sleep during their daily sleep period. These symptoms may be experienced by many shift workers. It has been suggested in some studies that about 30% of night shift workers doze off about once a week during work and about 50% report falling asleep while commuting home from work. These symptoms, however, are greatest in intensity and frequency, with an inability to adequately function, in shift work disorder subjects.

For your healthcare provider to confirm a diagnosis of shift work disorder, certain criteria must be fulfilled (see Question 15). Shift work disorder is considered a circadian rhythm sleep-wake disorder affecting people working either in permanent or rotating shifts (that is, working outside the traditional, normal working hours) whose schedule overlaps within their regular sleep period. During shift work, the workers have difficulty limiting light exposure to the appropriate time of day and hence have difficulty adapting to the new schedule. Light exposure shifts the body's rhythms to an earlier or later time depending on the time of exposure (see Question 20). Many of the other symptoms experienced by people with shift work disorder are secondary to excessive sleepiness or insomnia. **Excessive sleepiness** is considerd to be falling asleep in inappropriate places and under inappropriate circumstances, fatigue, inability to concentrate, and an impairment of motor skills and thinking. **Insomnia**

The two most important complaints in shift work disorder are excessive sleepiness in working hours and an inability to fall asleep or initiate sleep during their daily sleep period.

Excessive sleepiness

Having trouble staying awake enough to do the things you usually do.

Insomnia

The inability to obtain an adequate amount or quality of sleep to function efficiently during daytime.

is considered to be based on the following symptoms: difficulty falling asleep, frequent awakenings, non-refreshing sleep, inadequate hours of sleep, fatigue, irritability, lack of concentration, anxiety, and sometimes depression and forgetfulness.

Q14. How common is shift work disorder?

The exact **prevalence** of shift work disorder is unclear. Researchers think it may be as high as 10% (14.1% for the permanent night shift and 8.1% for rotating shift workers) of shift workers between 18 and 65 years. Considering that night and rotating shift workers comprise 6.4% of all workers, this translates into about 1% of the working population in the U.S. with shift work disorder. This is much less than the clinical estimate of 2% to 5% of the population cited by the International Classification of Sleep Disorders, Edition 2 (ICSD-2). In a recent study involving "swing" shifts (12 hour shifts lasting for two weeks, with one week of night shift followed by one week of day shift) among workers living continuously on sea-based oil platforms amongst the Norwegian off-shore oil industry, the prevalence of shift work disorder was estimated to be 23.3%, which is relatively high and could be explained by the specific working conditions on the oil rigs. Further research is needed to accurately determine prevalence.

Prevalence

The total number of cases of a disease in a given population at a specific time.

Q15. How do healthcare providers make a diagnosis of shift work disorder?

Healthcare providers generally follow the clinical diagnostic criteria (guidelines) established by the American Academy of Sleep Medicine listed in the ICSD-2. These criteria include the following: 1) patients must have significant insomnia or excessive sleepiness that interferes with functioning and is associated with a work schedule that overlaps the usual sleep period; 2) symptoms must be associated with a shift work schedule over the course of at least one month;

3) misalignment between the body clock and environmental clock manifested by loss of a normal sleep-wake pattern has been documented by sleep log or diary, and laboratory or home sleep recordings (see Question 17); and 4) sleep disturbance is not explained by another sleep disorder; a medical, neurological or psychiatric disorder; medication use; or substance abuse disorder.

If you are a shift worker who experiences excessive sleepiness or lack of non-restorative sleep that interferes with your ability to function at work or meet family and social obligations, you should contact your healthcare provider, who may then refer you to a sleep specialist for an accurate diagnosis. This is important for proper management and prevention of potential adverse consequences of shift work disorder.

Q16. Does shift work disorder affect every shift worker and if not, why not?

Not every shift worker will suffer from a true diagnosis of shift work disorder that satisfies all the diagnostic criteria (see Question 13). The reasons for this are complicated. For instance, there are certain risk factors that may predispose some people to developing shift work disorder, but not others. Two important factors are 1) different people have a different tolerance level for shift work, and 2) workers have different coping mechanisms. Some people can adapt to shift work and cope with the altered sleep-wake schedule better than others and the reasons for this are unclear. However, it may be genetic. The other factors predisposing to shift work disorder include pre-existing medical and psychological illnesses, lack of support from family and friends, and increasing age. All the factors listed in Table 1 also contribute to this predisposition. **Comorbid** (coexisting) sleep disorders, such as sleep apnea, restless legs syndrome, and prior history of insomnia, may also trigger the onset of shift work disorder. Each of us has a diurnal preference or chronotype, meaning that some people function best in the evening and so go to sleep later

Comorbid

The presence of one or more disorders (or diseases) in addition to a primary disease or disorder.

while others function best in the morning and go to bed earlier. However, this difference has not been consistently found to determine who develops shift work disorder.

Bindi writes:

I am a polysomnographic technologist (overnight sleep technician) and shortly after starting a rotating shift from day to night six months ago I started having sleep problems. I have been working two nights (Sunday and Monday from 7 pm to 7 am) and two days (Thursday and Friday from 8 am to 3:30 pm) a week. When I work nightshifts, the next day I have difficulty sleeping in the daytime. I barely get 3–4 hours of sleep even though my bedroom is very dark, with no telephone in the room. Later in the day I feel tired, fatigued, irritable, and agitated. When I go to work at night I am tired, but the excitement of learning and taking care of the patients prevents me from falling asleep during work.

When I come home in the morning after night shifts, it is very difficult for me to drive because of fatigue and sleepiness, but I manage the short distance of my commute by opening the windows and listening to loud music on the radio. My sleep log (for two weeks) attests to these symptoms affecting my sleep and mood during this shift work. I do not have a problem sleeping at night after my day shifts.

Q17. How does a healthcare provider approach a patient with shift work disorder?

First and foremost, your healthcare provider will confirm a diagnosis of shift work disorder and will look for associated medical, neurological, and psychiatric diseases, as well as primary sleep disorders (for example, sleep apnea, narcolepsy, restless legs syndrome, chronic insomnia, or other circadian rhythm sleep disorders), which might impact the symptoms of shift work disorder. Your provider will need to obtain a complete history, which includes a 24-hour sleep history, as well as medical, psychiatric, neurological, drug and alcohol, past and family histories. A physical examination is then performed to look for evidence of some of the other disorders as stated above. For confirmation of shift work disorder, your healthcare provider will pay close attention to the ICSD-2 diagnostic criteria (see Question 13). You may be given a sleep log or diary to establish your sleep-wake pattern for the preceding two weeks. You may also be given some scales (see **Table 3**) to help gauge your level of sleepiness.

Table 3. Epworth Sleepiness Scale

	Scores*
1. Sitting and reading	_____
2. Watching television	_____
3. Sitting in a public place (e.g., a theater or a meeting)	_____
4. Sitting in a car as a passenger without a break	_____
5. Lying down to rest	_____
6. Sitting and talking to someone	_____
7. Sitting quietly after lunch without alcohol	_____
8. In a car, while stopped for a few minutes in traffic	_____

Scale to determine total scores:
0 = Would Never Doze
1 = A slight Chance of Dozing
2 = Moderate Chance of Dozing
3 = High Chance of Dozing

For example, in the Epworth Sleepiness Scale the patient rates eight situations on a scale of 0-3, with 3 indicating a situation in which chances of dozing off are highest. The maximum score is 24 and a score of 10 suggests the presence of excessive sleepiness. Your healthcare provider may then order a polysomnographic (PSG) study (discussed further on) during day sleep (in night shift workers) to confirm sleep initiation or maintenance difficulty and presence of non-restorative sleep as well as to exclude other primary sleep disorders (such as sleep apnea). Other useful tests are the multiple sleep latency test and actigraphy (discussed further on).

What is a PSGstudy?

A *polysomnography* (PSGstudy) is a recording of activities from many of your body systems and organs while you sleep. It is a painless procedure with no discomfort to the patient. No needles are used, and the subject will not receive any electrical shock. The person having the test is connected to sensors and wires to equipment that records the various body system activities. A typical recording registers the electrical activities of the brain (**electroencephalogram or EEG**), the muscles (**electromyogram, or EMG**), eye movements (**electrooculogram, or EOG**), heart rhythm (**electrocardiogram, ECG or EKG**), respiratory pattern, snoring, body position, and blood oxygen saturation.

Electrical activities of the brain are recorded by using three to ten channels of a polygraph. The polygraph is somewhat similar to a "lie detector" machine (polygraph test). Of course, a sleep study takes place in the sleep laboratory, and it records many more physiological characteristics than those studied during lie detector tests.

For EEG (brain activity) recording, electrodes or sensors (small, cup-shaped or flat disks measuring about 5 to 6 mm) are painlessly attached to the scalp with a special adhesive. The sensors are connected by wires to the amplifiers of the polygraph. The electrical activities generated on the surface of the brain are tiny currents that must be amplified before they can be recognized on the monitor of the computer; hence, an amplifier is an essential part of the polygraph. Data is recorded by a computer for later review by medical staff.

Electro-encephalogram

Records of the electrical activities of the brain.

Electromyogram

Records of the activities of the muscles.

Electrooculogram

Records of eye movement activity.

Electrocardiogram

Records of heart rhythm activity.

To record eye movements (EOG), surface disks are placed over the upper corner of one eye and the lower corner of the other eye. Electrical activities of the muscles (EMG) are routinely recorded by placing sensors over the chin and outer aspects of the upper legs below both knees. EEG, EOG, and EMG readings are used to identify the different sleep stages.

In most cases, a patient's respiration pattern is recorded by using three channels. A sensor is placed over the upper lip below the nose to record airflow through the nose and mouth. A band across the chest and another band across the abdomen register respiratory (breathing) effort by recording chest and abdominal efforts for each inhalation and exhalation. In the most common type of sleep apnea, the airflow channels recording the activities from the sensors placed below the nose show no activity or markedly reduced activity, whereas the channels registering chest and abdominal movements continue to show effort or are deflected in opposite directions, indicating obstruction in the upper airway passage near the back of the tongue.

The amount of oxygen being carried in the patient's blood is recorded throughout the night by a finger clip. The finger clip registers changes in the color of hemoglobin (blood pigment); the color, which is shown on a monitor by a number (for example, 90% to 100% in a normal person), indicates blood oxygen saturation (oxygen is carried in the hemoglobin of the red blood cell). In patients with sleep apnea, the oxygen saturation of the blood falls below 90% when the breathing (airflow) stops.

To record snoring, a small microphone is attached over the front of the neck. Body position during sleep is monitored through a position sensor over the shoulder. The degree of sleep apnea is worse when a person lies on his or her back. In a routine recording, one channel is used to record electrical signals of the heartbeat (electrocardiogram) via sensors or the electrodes placed over the upper chest.

After placement of all sensors, the connecting wires are gathered into a bundle and attached to the board next to the patient. This board is then connected by wires going through the walls or the ceiling of the bedroom to the main polygraphic machine or computer in an adjacent room, where the technician will monitor a paperless recording and make necessary adjustments to obtain an optimal recording. If any of the electrodes (sensors and detectors) are disturbed, the technician will enter the patient's room and reposition the sensor so that it accurately records the data. The technician will also watch the video if such a recording is used (most laboratories generally also use video recording to observe any abnormal movements and behavior during sleep).

To begin the process, the patient will come to the laboratory at a specified time; in the case of a night shift worker it will likely be in the morning around 8 am. The technician explains the procedure to the patient and tries to set the patient at ease. Correctly placing the connections, preparing the machine, and explaining the procedure generally takes one to two hours. The technician then turns the lights off and asks the person to get ready to sleep. If the patient must get up in the middle of sleep to visit the bathroom, the bundle of wires can be easily disconnected from the machine and clipped to the patient's pajamas or nightwear, then reconnected again on returning to bed. At the end of the session (usually after 7–8 hours of recording) the technician will turn the lights on and remove the electrodes. The patient is then ready to go home unless he or she is scheduled to have a multiple sleep latency study to evaluate for sleepiness at night during work hours. PSG findings in shift work disorder consist of reduced total duration of sleep, usually 5–6 hours instead of the normal 7 1/2 to 8 hours; reduced sleep efficiency (expressed as the ratio of total sleep hours divided by total time in bed calculated in percent); decreased non-rapid eye movement Stage 2 sleep (major sleep stage occupying about 55% in normal individuals); and decreased dream stage or rapid eye movement sleep.

What is an MSLT?

A multiple sleep latency test (MSLT) is a test to assess the severity of sleepiness. In people working traditional hours, MSLT is performed during daytime following an overnight PSG study. In night shift workers, however, this test is performed at night to evaluate for excessive sleepiness during working hours. An MSLT is performed every two hours for four to five recordings, and each recording lasts as long as 20 minutes. For example, in night shift workers the test can be performed at 10 pm, 12 am, 2 am, 4 am, and 6 am. The electrical activities of the brain (EEG), chin muscles (EMG), and eye movements (EOG) are recorded during the 20-minute test. Patients are asked to refrain from drinking coffee and smoking during the day. Following an explanation of the test, the technician turns the lights off and asks the patient to lie down and try to go to sleep. In between the tests, the patient must stay awake and read, walk around, or watch television, but must not fall asleep; otherwise, the significance of the findings will remain questionable.

Sleep latency

The amount of time it takes to fall asleep.

The sleep specialist looks for two findings in the MSLT: **sleep latency**, which is the amount of time it takes the patient to fall asleep (as determined by the changes in brain wave activity) after the lights are turned off; and the presence of sleep-onset rapid eye movements (the dream stage of sleep that occurs within 15 minutes of falling asleep). An average sleep latency time is then calculated from the times that were recorded in each nap study. Any sleep latency of eight minutes or less is considered excessive sleepiness. An average sleep latency between eight and ten minutes indicates mild sleepiness and more than ten minutes is considered normal sleep latency.

PSG and MSLT recordings are not included in the formal diagnostic criteria for shift work disorder (see Question 13). In fact, there is no conclusive information about what the normal daytime PSG and nighttime MSLT recordings should be for shift workers without shift work disorder, thus these tests have limited diagnostic usefulness. These tests can help determine if other sleep disorders are present.

Another laboratory test which may be useful to show circadian disruption (a mismatch between the internal body clock and environmental time) is an **actigraphy recording**. Actigraphy involves wearing a watch-like device on the wrist or ankle to monitor activities of the body resulting from body movements—the **actigraph** is a motion detector. Presumably, we lie relatively immobile during sleep so the device should register few movements, whereas during wakefulness the actigraph records excessive body movements. In this way, an actigraph indirectly estimates the amount of sleep and wakefulness as well as the time of sleep starts and stops. The recording is important in patients with circadian rhythm sleep disorders, which cause them to experience difficulty in getting to sleep at the right time. Actigraphy recordings obtained over a two-week period in patients with shift work disorder may objectively document circadian disruptions showing reversal of sleep-wake rhythm, evidence of excessive sleepiness during working hours at night, and periods of wakefulness during day sleep episodes.

The next step is for your healthcare provider to help you minimize shift work related distress and treat the two major symptoms of sleep-wake disorder, namely insomnia and excessive sleepiness. The two primary goals of treatment are to 1) realign your internal body clock with the external altered sleep schedule by employing non-pharmacological (behavioral) countermeasures (so that your body adapts to the shift work schedule) and 2) symptomatic treatment to improve sleep and maintain wakefulness. To be most effective, treatment should combine behavioral, circadian, and pharmacological therapies.

Actigraphy recording

Continuously monitors body movement during periods of sleep and wakefulness with a special device called an actigraph.

Actigraph

A motion detector that records body motion through a watch-like device that is worn on the non-dominant wrist or ankle.

Q18. What are non-pharmacological countermeasures to treat shift work disorders?

Non-pharmacological countermeasures are aimed at improving the quality and quantity of sleep, lifestyle and healthy behaviors, and the practice of good sleep hygiene. All shift workers should follow good sleep hygiene practices. **Table 4** lists some commonsense measures that will minimize the adverse effects of shift work and strengthen coping mechanisms. It is important for shift workers to keep a consistent sleep-wake schedule, even on days when they do not work (this may be difficult due to family and social obligations and long-standing habits but it is important to follow the schedule consistently). Your home sleeping environment should help you fall asleep. Therefore, day sleepers should turn off all phone ringers (including cell phones) and darken the room by using heavy drapes and curtains. Educate family, friends, and neighbors about the importance of your uninterrupted sleep and encourage them not to disturb you. Ask callers to leave voice mail messages, put up "Do Not Disturb" signs on your bedroom or main door, and consider using a white noise machine to maintain a quiet environment. Following are some general recommendations specifically related to shift work: limit the duration and number of shifts in a row (for example, not more than three nights in a row); try to avoid rotating shifts, especially counterclockwise rotation or at least limit this rotation to no more than one rotating shift a week; avoid extended work hours including excessive overtime; arrange for short breaks during work hours; avoid exposure to light in the morning during the commute home from work and use sunglasses or goggles; avoid long commutes in the morning to minimize the chance of an accident and to have sufficient hours in the morning for sleep.

It is important for shift workers to keep a consistent sleep-wake schedule, even on days when they do not work.

Table 4

Sleep Hygiene Measures
• Keep a regular sleep-wake schedule, even on weekends or days off
• Sleep the amount needed to feel rested
• Avoid napping during the daytime
• Do not watch television, listen to loud music, or plan the next day's activities while in bed
• Avoid caffeinated beverages (coffee, tea, cola, hot chocolate) before bedtime
• Avoid alcohol near bedtime
• Avoid smoking, especially in the evening
• Do not go to bed hungry
• Adjust the bedroom environment
• Exercise regularly for at least 20 minutes, but do not exercise close to bedtime

Certain strategies for day sleep and napping are important countermeasures. To increase the amount of time you sleep (maximize sleep duration), a second sleep episode in the late afternoon or early evening for 1 to 1 1/2 hours ("**prophylactic naps**") has been shown to decrease accidents and improve wakefulness and performance. Short naps from 20 to 30 minutes, if possible, during shift work will improve wakefulness at work and improve performance. Longer naps (more than 30 to 40 minutes) may cause some degree of sleep inertia or "sleep drunkenness" (that is, a short period of persistent drowsiness and fatigue interfering with work). It is also important to include regular physical exercise as part of your efforts to improve sleep. If your sleep disturbance related to shift work persists, consult your healthcare provider or a sleep specialist (see Question 17).

Prophylactic naps

Naps taken as a precautionary measure to avoid sleep loss.

Shift Work Disorder

Q19. Are there medications for symptomatic treatment of excessive sleepiness or insomnia related to shift work or shift work disorder?

There are no medications that can "cure" shift work disorder. However, in addition to scheduled naps and other non-drug and behavioral therapies, there are some medications that are approved to treat the excessive sleepiness that occurs in some workers with shift work disorder. These wake-promoting agents must be prescribed by your healthcare provider after establishing the diagnosis of shift work disorder as discussed in Questions 3 and 17. Your healthcare provider will be in the best position to discuss whether these medications are right for you. Remember, these drugs treat only the symptoms and not shift work disorder itself.

There is a limited role for sleep medications to treat insomnia related to shift work and shift work disorder. Both over-the-counter and prescription sleep aids are available. Your healthcare provider or sleep specialist can help you determine whether a sleep aid is right for you. Simple lifestyle changes and good sleep hygiene habits may reduce the need for sleep medication (see Question 18 for daytime sleep hygiene recommendations).

Q20. What is the role of exposure to bright light in shift work disorder and how does it work?

Bright light therapy is a recommended non-drug therapy for certain circadian rhythm sleep disorders, including shift work disorder. The purpose of light therapy is to realign the internal body clock with the external or environmental time clock. Because the fundamental problem with shift work disorder is a mismatch between the internal body clock with imposed work and sleep-wake schedule, appropriately timed bright light therapy is a logical choice. Light exposure in the evening delays the rhythm (i.e., delays the sleep onset), whereas light exposure in the morning phase advances the rhythm (i.e., sleep onset occurs earlier in the evening). Therefore, bright light exposure in the early part of the night in night shift workers will delay their rhythm so that their sleep period can occur in the early morning and wakefulness will be maintained throughout the night. In addition, bright light also has an alerting effect that improves wakefulness, attention, memory, and concentration in night shift workers. A number of studies involving both actual and simulated shifts have shown improvement in performance, mood, and wakefulness.

There are no standard guidelines for the time of light exposure, the number of exposures, or the intensity of light. Generally, bright light with an intensity varying from 2,500 lux to 10,000 lux is used in the early part of the night. Sometimes it is given intermittently during the first 6 hours of work, lasting 15 to 20 minutes each time, separated by 45 minutes. This light therapy at night must be combined with avoidance of morning sunlight by wearing dark goggles or sunglasses during the commute home. Exposure to sunlight in the morning will phase advance the rhythm, thus counteracting the phase delay function of light exposure at night. Some studies have found an improvement in sleep duration and quality during the day following bright light therapy. Not all field studies supported the use of light therapy for shift workers. The American Academy of Sleep Medicine practice parameters, however, recommend such therapy. There may be some mild non-permanent side effects associated with bright light therapy such as headache, eye strain, irritability, and blurred vision. Subjects with retinopathies (diseases affecting the nerve cell layer in the back of the eye), those using photosensitizing medications (consult your healthcare provider to find out if you are using any photosensitizing medication), and those with bipolar disorder should not be given bright light therapy. One controversial but serious consideration is the possibility of increased risk of breast cancer in women as a result of suppression of melatonin by bright light (see Question 9).

Appendix

American Academy of Sleep Medicine (AASM)
2510 North Frontage Road
Darien, IL 60561
Telephone: 630-737-9700
www.aasmnet.org

The mission of the AASM is to promote sleep disorder medicine to members of the medical and paramedical professions as well as to the public. The organization is dedicated to supporting quality care for patients with sleep disorders, providing professional and public education on the issues, and encouraging and supporting research in sleep medicine.

National Center for Sleep Disorders Research (NCSDR)
2 Rockledge Center, Suite 7024
6701 Rockledge Drive, MSC7920
Bethesda, MD 20892-7920
Telephone: 301-435-0199
www.nhlbi.nih.gov/sleep

The NCSDR was established based on a 1993 recommendation by a Congressionally mandated national commission on sleep disorders research. This center is located within the National Heart, Lung, and Blood Institute of the National Institutes of Health (NIH) in Bethesda, Maryland. It supports research, education, and training in sleep and sleep disorders for all healthcare professionals. The center also participates in public awareness and education campaigns about sleep disorders. It works in collaboration with several federal agencies, including the NIH, the former Alcohol, Drug Abuse, and Mental Health Administrations, and the Departments of Defense, Transportation, and Veterans Affairs.

National Sleep Foundation (NSF)
729 Fifteenth Street, NW, 4th Floor
Washington, DC 20005
Telephone: 202-347-3471

The NSF produces valuable brochures dealing with sleep and sleep disorders, promotes public education (particularly about driving, fatigue, and sleepiness as well as important sleep disorders), and periodically organizes Gallup polls dealing with sleep and sleep difficulties.

Restless Legs Syndrome (RLS) Foundation
1610 14th Street, NW, Suite 300
Rochester, MN 55901
Telephone: 507-287-6465
www.rls.org

The RLS Foundation was established by patients suffering from RLS in 1990 and is guided by an RLS scientific advisory board and a medical advisory board. Its mission is to support patients with RLS and their families. The RLS Foundation also provides information to educate health care providers about RLS and sponsors research intended to find better treatments and, eventually, a definitive cure. Members (patients with RLS) receive newsletters with valuable information about the disease and support groups throughout the country.

Glossary

Actigraph: a motion detector that records body motion through a watch-like device that is worn on the non-dominant wrist or ankle.

Actigraphy Recording: Continuously monitors body movement during periods of sleep and wakefulness with a special device called an actigraph.

Cataplexy: A sudden loss of muscle tone and strength without loss of consciousness.

Chronic Sleep Disturbance: The inability to obtain sufficient amount of good quality sleep resulting in daytime sleepiness.

Circadian Rhythm: Internal body clock representing a 24-hour cycle.

Comorbid: The presence of one or more disorders (or diseases) in addition to a primary disease or disorder.

Electrocardiogram (ECG or EKG): Records of heart rhythm activity.

Electroencephalogram (EEG): Records of the electrical activities of the brain.

Electromyogram (EMG): Records of the activities of the muscles.

Electrooculogram (EOG): Records of eye movement activity.

Excessive Sleepiness: Having trouble staying awake enough to do the things you usually do.

Homeostatic Sleep Drive: The desire to sleep that gradually increases with prolonged wakefulness.

Insomnia: The inability to obtain an adequate amount or quality of sleep to function efficiently during daytime.

Narcolepsy: Chronic neurological sleep disorder characterized by overwhelming daytime drowsiness and sudden attacks of sleep.

Prevalence: The total number of cases of a disease in a given population at a specific time.

Prophylactic naps: Naps taken as a precautionary measure to avoid sleep loss.

Shift Work: Untraditional night or rotating between night and day work schedule.

Sleep paralysis: The inability to voluntarily move when falling asleep or waking up.

Sleep latency: The amount of time it takes to fall asleep.

Index

Index